ANDREW CARR

How HIIT changed my life

This book was professionally typeset on Reedsy.
Find out more at reedsy.com

Contents

Introduction

Welcome to How HIIT Changed My Life. My name is Andrew Carr and this is a brief true story about how interval training truly changed my life. I'm so excited to share with you this journey. My life was changed forever, for the better, in ways that I never dared dream and my hope is that one day your life will change as well.

You're probably thinking, this guy grew up with some holistic or athletic background. That couldn't be further from the truth. I grew up in Tennessee and was pretty much the average kid. I spent time playing video games, listening to music and getting outside of the house every chance that I got. I drank soda and ate whatever was in the house. I ate all of the junk food in the world. The only sports I played before middle school was some church league basketball. I was the most unathletic kid on the team. I was always the kid that was picked last for all the sports. I was skinny, couldn't think fast on my feet, couldn't catch very well and didn't have the size to overpower anyone.

Fast forward to middle school and I started running cross country, track and I even wrestled a little. I was never a starter on the wrestling team and I never placed or had any great results running. All I could ever say about running was that I just had the knack to not quit and run whatever length I was told to run.

In high school, after we'd moved across the state, I played football my freshman year and played baseball one fall. The highlights of my football career include getting put in for a play when our team was winning

52-0. I was the smallest kid on the team, went to every practice and practiced as hard as I could but I was never big, strong or fast enough to be a good athlete. The highlight of my baseball career was hitting a double one night when we were playing a team that wasn't nearly as good as us. That pitcher must have been as horrible as I was to let me get an extra base hit. Maybe God just felt sorry for me that day and let me get a lucky hit. Either way, I'll take it.

After my freshman year of high school, I didn't play any sports and started working odd jobs around my neighborhood cleaning up construction sites. Our neighborhood was brand new and we were one of the first families to move in. When I was working, I was the assistant of a guy named David. David, who I thought was pretty cool at the time, drove a Camaro, smoked cigarettes and had long hair. This was where I tried my first cigarette. David let me smoke one and the next thing you know, I'm saving my money to spend on cigarettes.

Then, I met a guy in our neighborhood who was a drummer in a local band. His mom kept cartons of cigarettes in her freezer and he'd give me packs whenever I wanted them. Strangely enough my parents never said anything to me about smoking. Neither of my parents smoked and were very religious. The first time I was caught smoking was when I climbed up in our attic to smoke one night and my parents could smell it. That was my sophomore year of high school.

During the summer between my sophomore and junior years of high school we moved to Georgia. I got a job working at the local grocery store as soon as my parents would let me. This afforded me the luxury to ride my bike to work and I could swing by the local convenience store and buy cigarettes on my way to work. I'd also get any of the broken packs of cigarettes that were lying around the grocery store.

This kept on for the remainder of high school and next thing you I'm headed to college. As you can imagine, my decision making didn't get any better. By this time in my life I was a full blown smoker. The next vice that got added to my rituals was drinking. My buddies and I would go to teen night at the local country club and have a few beers before we went. This progressed to drinking on the weekends when we weren't working, drinking after work and then drinking anytime we were able to hang out together.

When I finally turned 21 and was able to buy alcohol for myself, we were hanging out in the bars every night. We were in the clubs that we'd been going to on teen nights and the ones that we got into illegally. It was at this time that I met my future wife. She was one of the pretty girls in the bar that sold beer for tips. Goodness, did I give her a lot of money!!

She and I turned into drinking buddies and going to the bars every night after work. We got married, never had any kids, and partied every chance we got. I was smoking two packs of cigarettes every day (at least) and we were eating the cheapest and least healthy foods imaginable. All of our food came out of a box or a drive through window. There was absolutely nothing healthy about our lifestyles in any shape, form or fashion.

This pattern kept on for years until I'd had a couple of DUIs and she'd cheated on me and we decided to get a divorce. After my divorce, I moved into the city of Atlanta so that I could enjoy all the fun that the city had to offer. I partied every single chance that I possibly could. This led to another DUI and this time the consequences were stiff. I was put into the county's DUI court and forced to remain sober. For the first time in my life I saw the nature of my wrongs and the depth of all my poor decisions over the course of my life.

Let's make one thing clear before going any further. I do NOT take any pride in all of the poor decisions that I made. Drinking and driving is wrong. There's nothing good about it and I wish that I'd never done it. Thank God that I didn't kill anyone with my selfish and reckless actions. I'm giving you this backstory so that you can see the extent to which my life was in shambles when I decided to change my life.

Why I started training

Needless to say at this point in my life, I knew my life was in shambles. I had no drivers license. I had to take public transportation or ride my bicycle. The only bike I had was a heavy mountain bike that wasn't made for the streets of Atlanta. The first time that I rode my bike to the closest AA meeting, I thought I was going to die. Literally and figuratively I thought that my lungs were going to give out before my legs or body did.

This was the point that I started "training" and told myself that I was going to "get healthy". Little did I know what the future held. I called my brother, a successful chiropractor, to brag to him that I'd started running again and was "eating healthy". This is the point that he showed me that the founder of the running movement died from heart issues at age 52 and that my diet wasn't healthy at all. Seriously?! How could this be? Does this mean that everything that I'd seen on the television about what was healthy and what wasn't was wrong? How could this be true?

I'd quit drinking soft drinks. I could drink a gallon of soft drinks every day. I'd started drinking milk. That has to be healthy right? Not exactly. I was buying protein from the local Wal-Mart. That had to be good, right? Well, not exactly it seems.

It was at this point my brother told me about High Intensity Interval Training or HIIT for short. This, my friends, is exactly where the game began to change.

What is HIIT?

High Intensity Interval Training really isn't as intimidating as it sounds. My brother used to call it high intensity short duration workouts. All this means, in simple terms, is you workout hard for a brief period of time as hard as you can, rest and then do it again. It really is THAT simple. As a matter of fact, you can do this with any type of exercise!!

You're probably saying to yourself, wait a minute. Hold up. Stop. It can't be THAT easy. Actually it is. However, at the same time, it really isn't that easy. What I'm trying to say is that it's that simple but it isn't easy. Once again, the first time that I tried it I really did think I was going to die when it was over. The best part about it is, not only did I not die, but I felt AMAZING when it was all finished and couldn't wait to workout again the next day.

What I've learned about HIIT, is that it trains all of the systems in your body at the same time where other forms of workouts do not. Yes, running trains your lungs but it also releases cardiac stresses on your heart for extended periods of time and doesn't help build strong functional muscles across your entire body. Lifting heavy weights builds bigger muscles but it doesn't train your heart and lungs very well. HIIT trains your muscles building lean functional muscle and trains your lungs, heart and other organs at the same time.

HIIT not only builds lean muscle but it also is known to burn more calories, improve your metabolism, improve your cardiovascular health, increase your oxygen consumption, relieve your stress and increase your levels of human growth hormone. So you're probably asking yourself, why are these things important? Do all of these things really matter that much? They do matter that much!

As we all know, burning more calories that you intake will help in weight loss. So anyone that's overweight can appreciate this point. Science has even proven that interval training can increase your metabolism for up to 36 hours AFTER you finish working out. Increasing your oxygen consumption is much bigger than you realize at first. Not only does it help you breathe easier, but it also aids in fighting cells that can become cancerous. Otto Warburg, who discovered cancer, identified cancerous cells as cells that live in environments that were low in oxygen and acidic. When we oxygenate our blood, we put our bodies in position to fight against certain forms of cancers. I've not met anyone who isn't looking for some sort of stress relief in their life, so I'll leave this topic alone for now. Increasing human growth hormones in your body has been proven to help you fight the effects of aging and increase how many calories your body can burn.

So as you can see, just by doing a few short workouts, you can start changing the direction that your life is going. These changes won't immediately make you skinny or make you able to run a marathon right away, but with consistent training and paying attention to how you workout, you can do those things eventually.

So you're probably asking, ok, but who can do HIIT? The answer is simple, anyone! Yes, you can do HIIT today, no matter what shape you're physically in right now. You might be thinking I'm overweight, I already have heart issues, I have a bad knee, I can't even touch my toes or any other reason you can imagine. The beautiful thing about HIIT is that you can start today with any exercise that you can do. You might just be able to do a few jumping jacks or run in place for a little bit. You might only be able to do some shoulder presses with soup cans and not any heavy weight. All of that is perfect!!

The truth is that everyone's journey starts uniquely. Where you are at physically may be better or worse than where I was. You might be in a better or worse position than your spouse or even your children. It's ok! You're right where you need to be and you're the only person who knows what your body is capable of doing. So you can be the judge of how easy or complex your workouts can be. The fact remains, that when you start training, you immediately get the gift of a higher metabolism. You get the gift of giving your heart a natural stent. For those of you who don't know, a stent is what the doctors put in to open the veins and arteries around your heart during heart surgery. This makes the blood flow more easily. You give that to your heart naturally with HIIT. The best part is you don't have to go through surgery and heart problems to get it!

Where can you do HIIT?

This is truly one of the best benefits of HIIT! You don't need a gym membership or a bunch of equipment to get started on your life changing journey today. You can literally do HIIT anywhere you want to. When I first got sober I was sharing a tiny two bedroom house with someone. We didn't have a living room. All we had was two bedrooms, a shared bathroom and a shared kitchen. I began my HIIT journey in my bedroom with no equipment to workout with at all.

As you progress, you can certainly go to a gym if you'd like to and you can purchase accessories to enhance your workout along the way. Some of the places that I've done interval training are local parks, the college track close to my house, the street I live on, my bedroom, my garage, my driveway, under my deck, beside the pool,in a chiropractor's office, on the beach and in my backyard. The possibilities are literally endless. Anywhere you can find space and a little bit of time is perfect to workout with.

What do you need to do HIIT?

The number one thing you need to do HIIT is a great mindset. Like I said earlier, HIIT is simple but it's not easy. Having a positive mindset from the beginning will make all the difference in the world to your success.

Secondly, like I also stated earlier, you don't need any fancy equipment or location to do your workouts. This makes HIIT perfect for everyone that is looking for permanent life change. You can even use simple objects around your house as weights. I used soup cans once after someone recommended them to me and my shoulders were completely sore the next day thanks to just adding a little soup to the exercise.

Thirdly, you need just a little extra time. This step will make all the difference in your training. When you're putting your workouts together, take a few minutes and look up the proper form needed for the exercise that you choose. Maintaining good form through all of your workouts is imperative. It's better to do one good rep of an exercise than 40 bad reps. Your muscles will thank you and you'll see improvements at a much greater pace this way.

Fourth, in today's age of smartphones and tablets, you can download free HIIT timers that will help make working out SO much easier.

How do you do HIIT?

I'm sure you've been wondering, ok so exactly how do you do HIIT? HIIT is really simple. I'll break down my first workout for you. Essentially I exercised for 20 seconds and then I rested for 20 seconds. I did a different exercise for 20 seconds and then I rested for another 20 seconds. Then I repeated this same procedure for 4 more exercises. That completed 1 set. Then I did 3 more sets of the same 4 exercises. Essentially I exercised for 8 minutes and rested for 8 minutes.

I know you're probably thinking that it cannot be that hard. Trust me!! It was!! The secret to HIIT is doing those exercises as fast as you can and doing them with the best possible form. By the time that I'd reached the third and fourth sets my muscles were exhausted.

Having exhausted muscles isn't bad and it doesn't mean that you have to quit exercising. I told my brother about the workout that I'd done and how I'd slowed down on my last set and he gave me a piece of information that changed my world. He told me that you can modify exercises to make them easier and this enables you to keep working out hard. He told me that when my muscles were burnt out from push ups to start doing pushups on my knees. Then he told me that I could even do push ups on a wall.

You're probably thinking that's crazy. I was thinking that as well! He's right though, you can modify any exercise to make it easier so that when your muscles are fatigued you can still push your muscle to it's limit. I've modified countless exercises to make sure that I could still do the exercise. The results were astounding. Before you know it, I was modifying exercises to make them harder. This was when I knew that my body was starting to change and adapt to this new lifestyle.

Exercises

I've broken these exercises down into 3 categories. My goal for you, whatever your physical situation is, to be able to exercise and get started. Some of these exercises may be easier for some than others. You may have knee problems and need exercises that are easier on your knees, but you have a strong upper body. You are free to pick and choose from this list and modify the exercise, or the list of exercises, however you please. The following lists are just recommendations. They are by no means the complete list of exercises. This list was made to give you the freedom to do whatever exercises you can with the abilities you have. You're free to add and take away from these lists however you choose.

Beginner Exercises

- Arm Circles
- Standard push-up
- Plank
- Squat (Preacher's squat)
- Lunge
- Mountain Climbers
- Wall Sit
- Calf Raise

- Good Mornings
- Crunch
- Bicycles
- Shoulder Press (no weight or light weight)
- Lat Pull Downs (using light weight bands)
- Bicep Curls (using light weight)
- Tricep Curls (using light weight)

Intermediate Exercises

- Shoulder Bridge
- Step Ups
- Burpee
- Inch Worm
- Tuck Jump
- Bear Crawl
- Stair climb with bicep curls
- Clock Lunge
- Curtsy Lunge
- Squat reach and jump
- Contralateral Limb Raise
- Donkey Kick
- Tricep Dip
- Diamond Push-ups
- Boxer

Expert Exercises

- Handstand Push-ups
- Judo Push-ups
- Superman

- Chair Pose Squat
- Squat Reach and Jump
- Lunge Jump
- Pistol Squats

The key to all of these exercises, and I'll say it again for those in the back, do as many reps as possible with the best possible form. Always remember, that you can add and take away from all these exercises as needed. You can add a weight vest, dumbbells, resistance bands (10/10 recommend), soup cans and anything else you can dream up to make these exercises harder for just a set or two.

Life Changes

So you're probably wondering, how exactly did the gift of HIIT change my life. Well, the changes in my life were astronomical. Every single area of my life changed. My physical, mental, home and work lives changed for the best in every way imaginable.

Physically I went from a two plus pack a day smoker to running obstacle course races competitively on the weekend. I have run races all over the east coast of the United States. I started with Spartan races in the southeast. A Spartan race is an obstacle course race that makes you use every muscle in your body. There are many different lengths of races from about 3-5 miles all the way up to ultra marathon lengths. For those of you that don't know, an ultra marathon is any race over 26.2 miles.

My very first obstacle course race was about 15 miles (I had no idea the distance before I signed up and paid for it) and about 30 obstacles. If you cannot complete an obstacle there is a penalty of 30 burpees. A burpee is an exercise that's known for how bad it sucks. It's a push-up into a jump squat that burns your body and your lungs. What's even more crazy is that, not only did I run the 15 mile version, but the next day I ran the 10 mile version the next day. Total transparency here, my time the next day was just as long as my time the day before. I was so mentally and physically exhausted that a shorter race took the same amount of time as the long race the day prior. But guess what? I DID IT!! I finished!!

This was a huge turning point in my life. I realized that the guy who couldn't ride a bike one mile (mostly downhill) to an AA meeting a few months prior, could now run a half marathon obstacle course race. Why is this so you ask? Well, when you train HIIT style, not only are you training your muscles but you're also training your lungs and all of your body's other systems at the same time. This type of training takes your body to a state where you're lacking oxygen and causing you to breath harder and heavier than you would by just running or lifting weights. This puts your body in an anaerobic state where your body is lacking oxygen you're training yourself at about 80-90%. This training causes you to build endurance. Little did I ever know when I started this that I'd build endurance.

About 10 months later I ran a race in Vermont. It was an ultra Spartan Race. This race was over 26.2 miles and 60+ obstacles. Not only was this race over a marathon with over 60 obstacles, but it was through the mountains of Killington, Vermont. They had us running up and down double black diamond ski slopes. It sounds intimidating doesn't it?! It was intimidating. On top of all of that, this race in particular had the highest did not finish (DNF) rate of all the Spartan races. This race had a 75% failure rate.

Before I started out on this race, I talked to my family on the phone and my sister-in-law's exact words were "don't die please". She was well aware of my past and all my poor decisions. She knew exactly how hard this would be for me. It was during this race that I realized another benefit that HIIT had given me. It has given me much greater mental strength as well.

Mentally

Because I'd learn to train my body to the point of exhaustion and done with great regularity, I'd trained my brain to be able to persevere through harder circumstances. Like when I was on the last climb of the race at 7:00pm, watching the sunset over the Green Mountains in Vermont, my legs were absolutely on fire. I'd take 15-20 steps up this incredibly steep mountain, then I'd turn around and walk backwards up the mountain to move the stresses on my legs. Instead of my quadriceps burning now my calves were burning. Then I'd change and walk normally up the mountain. I did this alternating until I made it to the top of the mountain.

When I was running through the trails in the dark at the bottom of the mountain, just me and my headlamp, I wanted to quit. It was getting cold. It was late. I started thinking that I might not make it. Then in my head I remembered everyone that was cheering for me. My friends that I'd made online and at other races, my brother and sister-in-law, my young nephews, my parents, my cousins and all my extended family were all cheering me on when I left home for this race. In my darkest moments I told myself that I was doing this so that I could physically be able to spend more time with them. That kept me going in ways that words simply cannot express.

When I got to the last of the long hard obstacles, I'd realized that I really could do anything. As I picked up my log to carry up to the next pole of the ski lift, I realized that if I could just get through this obstacle in time I'd finish the race. That same will and determination that I'd carved through trying to get to the end of my interval training got me through that obstacle. I finished that obstacle 23 seconds ahead of the time cut. The course judge was watching his watch and telling all of us when he was cutting the course off for safety.

Sure enough I was right!! After that obstacle, it was a pretty easy end of the race with easier obstacles and I finished the race 15 minutes before I ran out of time. I had just finished the Killington Ultra the first time out. A former two pack a day smoker and recovering alcoholic just finished the Killington Ultra the first time out!! Did it take me 14 hours and 45 minutes? Yes it sure did. But this guy didn't get kicked off the course. This guy didn't quit.

Home Life

Some of the biggest changes in my life that were brought about by all of this were in my home life. I went from being winded and not being able to breathe when I worked on my house or in my yard, to doing all of the things around the house with relative ease. Heck, I even painted the back deck at my parents house in the middle of August on a weekend. When I first told my father that I was going to do it for him on the weekend, he laughed uncontrollably. When I was finished that Sunday night, he couldn't believe that I had the endurance and the mental strength to do what I'd done. I didn't think that it was all that crazy until I realized how much the sun takes out of you.

The thing that has surprised me most about all of this was how my diet changed. Because I was working out in a manner that asked a lot from my body, I started giving my body the things that it needed to operate at its best. I quit drinking soda and sweet tea every where I went and started drinking more water. I quit drinking as much dairy (I LOVE whole milk). I started drinking more coconut and almond milk. I started actually eating vegetables. When I learned the value of greens and the amount of nutrients in them, I started consuming more greens than ever. I replaced my vitamins from the grocery store with quality vitamins. These changes didn't happen fast or all at once. They were all small changes that eventually led to greater results.

I'd never ask you to make all of these changes all at once. That is way too overwhelming to consider. My hope is that, as you go through your journey, you'll start looking into the benefits of what you put into your body. My hope is that you'll choose life and health over the immediate benefit of heavily processed foods. My hope is that you'll begin to see all of these small decisions as decisions that will help you to spend more time with those you love and care about. Maybe you'll add a year, or two, or five or ten or even twenty to your life. That'll enable you to see more kids, grandkids, graduations, football games, soccer games, baseball games and enjoy more the things in life that you want to do.